SHORT STORIES & POETRY

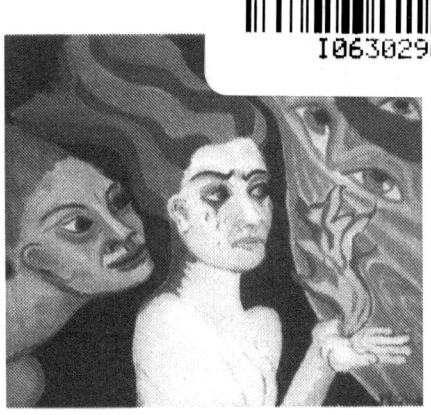

I0630296

BY MAUREEN OLIVER

'One million people commit suicide every year.'
The World Health Organization

MAUREEN OLIVER

Published by
Chipmunkapublishing
PO Box 6872
Brentwood
Essex CM13 1ZT
United Kingdom

http://www.chipmunkapublishing.co.uk

Proof-read by Anna Gomez

Cover image by Maureen Oliver.

Three Women and a Mirror

The Room

Three white walls, one interrupted by a window – the other wall is a mirror floor to ceiling. A bed. A bookshelf. A figure on the bed still asleep under a yellow quilt. The floor is heaped with discarded clothes, a stereo, books, and an empty wine bottle. Notes and messages are pinned to the walls –a pencil drawing, a child's scribble, a coloured bead necklace hangs on a nail.

Early morning – the light in the room shifts and pales into shades of pink and grey, watery sunlight fills the room. The mirror reflecting the sleeping figure, now stirring slightly, eyes moving, slight sounds. The mirror darkens as a cloud outside the window, beyond sight, passes in front of the rising sun. Shadows deepen, lighten again, but remain.

Three reflected shapes appear, vague, but definable as women.

The figure on the bed is awake, eyes wide, looking, looking, searching the mirror as the shapes form into three clear images staring dumbly through the glass, pressing against the glass as if seeking to enter the room, hands pushing in but then fading – fading into the familiar reflections of inanimate objects.

J is the figure on the bed. J is still sitting scanning the mirror. Only the stereo, books, clothing, a wine bottle, messages on the wall and J are in the room.

Annie, Sylv, Mole.

Annie is awakened by the children and is sitting up in her purple and green and red room thinking about cornflakes and last night's washing up. Then she remembers J and is at once bitter and sad, before she remembers to laugh, then climbs out of bed and dresses in the half-light.

Sylv is awakened by the shifting of her husband's arm, which is uncomfortably lodged in the small of her back. She rubs her eyes sleepily and looks out at a pale blue sky. A crash sends her scudding downstairs to her child, who is standing forlornly amidst broken glass and spilled milk. "Want a drink Mummy". While wielding the mop, she is suddenly uncomfortably reminded of J. Dreams a second. The noise of her husband searching for clean underpants breaks into her reverie. A feeling of sucking mud around her, swallowing her, suffocating, getting into her eyes, her throat. The swinging of the mop exerts a controlling composing rhythm and her mind clears into the usual comforting patterns – safe again.

Mole is still really half asleep when she becomes conscious of dampness around her caused by the soggy presence of her younger daughter. She creeps blindly out of bed, down the stairs and into the bathroom. While brushing her teeth, and looking at the vague puffy-eyed reflection in the mirror, she thinks of J and experiences a faint dizziness before remembering she has to make breakfast and feed the cat.

After a time J rises from the bed, the yellow quilt slides half way to the floor gently. J turns to the mirror in which the yellow quilt slides gently to the floor, J walks toward the mirror, towards J, until J is facing J, hands touching hands through the thin glass, fingertips nearly touching, bright eyes staring into bright glassy eyes. More time passing, sunlight is filling the still room – both still rooms – until the figures separate, the hands unlinking, turning back toward the bed, then J sits staring thoughtfully into the glass – reflection into reflection.

Sylv

Here I am washing the dishes again, taking the pie out of the oven, it's so hot and fresh for his dinner, waiting for his key to turn in the lock, watching the summer sky turn to pink and flush magenta and gold at the horizon – how beautiful, how precious, precious. Oh, I hear the child moan in his sleep – otherwise the little house is so still... I can sense its breathing among all the other silent houses in the neat suburban street. It's confusing, sometimes the face of my lover appears to demand more than I can give, refuses to accept what I can offer, demanding, demanding – they always take, but what could he give me – his love? Oh no, I must have comfort, support, a life to look forward to, protection from the dark, from the monsters of cruelty that pace my life with measured tread, someone to guard me, to cherish me, like my father, yes, him, my father, so strong yet kind – not like she – the mother...

How pretty was my lover, his eyes of warm,

promising blue; sensual mouth, warm tasting; and the touch of gentle fingertips that said love to me. Means stars, heavens, passion, depths, crimson seas... Yet as he spoke, clutching my hand, seducing my mind with those eyes, I saved myself from the anguish of commitment by tracing invisible beautiful patterns on the shape of his face. A triangle, another, a star – that line joined to that line and that – and I was safe. The potatoes are burning...

His love lied anyway, Mole knew, all the while he depended on Annie's mothering arms and the grip of Mole's floundering embrace – false friends – false lover. I could take the triangle of Mole and him and me. Seemed right, seemed almost natural, the competition was stimulating – but Annie shattered the equilibrium. Now I cannot think of her without a burning pain under my skull. Is ho so weak then that she could just reach out and take him? She wrapped him like a boy child in her great soft bed – taught him her ways, decided to have him, then finally derided him for his baby tears and craving her approval – why?

The question's hopeless, the sky is darkening, and husband is late, dinner spoiled. Husband cried too. It grows cold. I could not leave the home – the bed might be velvet and the passion burn sweet – but the cruel teeth of the world would be too close. If only one like my father…

Annie

Again and again the brain slips into that dark, warm, soft place of blessed emptiness – so far, so far from the cruelty of the clashing and violent colours that jar my singed eyeballs with consciousness of the bitter reality of the grey windswept plains of my life. Again and again I have felt promised gardens flowering fruitful, happy with children, smiling rosy brown and naked under the ever rising sun filling the vast horizon of my paradise – and some kind of a man who would blot out the pain and the dull screams of memory that echo and reecho across the ashes of those vast plains under a purple sky.

The thunder rolls, the rain sleets down upon the basement window, it is getting darker. The children are asleep at last. Tonight no man of warmth to bring me comfort – I had to drive J away. The threat of him, the curse of his clawing affection would have torn me apart piece by piece, then, stepping over the blood and spilt guts and brains he would smile and blithely go out without even a backward glance. Poisonous hopes die now. Well, men are all just different faces of the same thing, aren't they? The fat wanker who followed Mole and I down the King's Road was as much a man as J. They disguise it in love, they disguise it in blue-eyed innocence – yet there he was making love to me and crying over Sylv, and Mole crying to me for him – how much do they think my shoulders can bear? Too much pain.

Send me a man who is brave and strong, who can face the daggers of my mad eyes. Thunder again, the sound of the rain – sea-thrash to my troubled mind, stormy waters. J threatened me with his falseness, his mocking warmth. Now I feel demonic laughter mocking me and I see the treachery in his weeping eyes – the eyes that charmed, enchanted me – that had power spun from a devilish source. He told me how he lay sleeping and dreamed of being paralyzed while the stinging buzz of cruelty held him fast. He is possessed. I got hurt, scratches on the festering wounds, the open sores of broken loves – tears came at first – don't cry no more, tears gone, all finished.

Now I clear dirty cups from the table, place them in the sink, open the bedroom door and peer at the sleeping children lost in the sweet scent of their dreams, and go into my purple room and sit down – roll a cigarette, pour a glass of cider. Got to laugh though – fucking ridiculous! I can see the grey wolf slinking, his tongue lolling disguising the yellow teeth, into my room, the rank, foul smell, he mounts my bed. Then I see only the dreaming blue-eyed child man seeking the warmth of my body. This experience is a cynical joy like the over-ripe fruit on the market stall I poke with weary fingers while the children fret and whine on a hot, hot cobalt skied dusty day.

Now I am free – inches from my face a door opens into the enchanted garden, if only I can open my eyes… If only I can open my eyes I can see.

Mole

Tangled grasses, red sky above, throbbing yellow, leafy green trees soaring; feeling burning lust, wanting sweet love. Sticky-fingered mesh of friendship and jealously – J at centre, confuser or confused, doesn't matter now, does it?

Lying by his side feeling the warmth, eyes closing as in sleep but still not sleeping, holding him – somehow the grasp is torment. Annie felt malignancy in the warmth of his snake charming eyes – I don't, do I? And does he really exist save in the fever of my wishes and hopes? If I look up suddenly while he is unaware, will he still be there? The time that is now, the time I have him, that he has me, now that he has let the others go, that I have him, that he… this time I feel is not real time, is like a dreaming time, more than that, like stepping over the brink of the real time into a time that is not quite a dream but a different real world – like I slipped through the silver threads of this, whatever it is, time, into the parallel of a new or old world. Enough, what of the game that Annie and I played and are playing?

The mirror tinted blue and grey, river and rain, rain and river.

They alighted from the red bus at Westminster Bridge with the river green sludge at one side and the rain sheeting down between and around them. As they trod the Embankment, the railings pulsed behind the green oval of Annie's face – slightly turned towards her own. Purple and black striped glow around the oval with the staring yellow eyes and the, could that be mocking, smile? They walked to the Tate Britain, smiling quietly at one another, and the depths of the sky glowered as their feet rung hollow sounds on the pavement.

Looking at pictures, fairy images, madness and gentility and Blake and demons and torments of the damned. The air struck them fresh again outside, they were changed, otherness settled like soft dust, the rain was falling silently and the passing people stared through pinkly puffy faces and smiled sharp toothed – minds put out tentacles into the greenery-grey decay of city wrapped around arches and columns; the familiarity of the buildings masked by the waving of trees – the foliage waving. And, oh, the crowds of wild-eyed wanderers – how they sparked malice in the soul here on the smoky street, the air a seething gas poisoning the intricate passages of mind and body.

When we left the bus at Kennington the driver asked where we were going. Only here and now and we smiled secretly at one another and began to play the game.

Shops were dark and closed, the cake shop filled with bleeding meat, the houses in the familiar street had been demolished – replaced with endless corrugated iron fencing.

She stopped when I stopped; she stood under a tree, as did I. We laughed without joy and smiled knives – the daggers of her eyes were chrome yellow and she turned away into a tunnel. I hesitated. The tunnel was too dark; I hid behind a pillar. A space of time. I looked out. She was peering at me from behind another pillar – eyes piercing yellow light. I walked on, she was beside me, I stopped again; she stopped. The rain wet the skin, soft beneath sodden clothes. Chilling breath. Her eyes caught mine – smiling. The street was deserted save for us two. I hid behind a wall – when I turned she was smiling at me. I felt my head split into cool glass pieces stained blues and reds. Shattered splinters cut the wall of my face into a smile – idiot smile. Walking on I could not, could not – and the rain falling. I had lost the game.

The rain falling on the mirror had flecked it with watery blue, which the rainbows passing through had coloured. The hot sunlight pouring through the window touches J's hair with gold as he crosses the room again.

As J sleeps in the almost complete darkness of the little room, the mirror reflecting the mirror reflecting him seems to glow with a dim light.

Sylv sits cross-legged in the little garden of her neat house and talks endlessly to Mole of J. She speaks while mentally constructing a pentacle on the wide whiteness of Mole's face. Holding in her hand the gold St Christopher that J always wore round his neck she says, " As long as I have this I have some power over him…" She passes it to Mole and Mole presses it hard into her palm. "It is him", says Mole, handing it back. The sun is warm in the garden and they have been eating salad. It is very still, only insects buzzing on the roses – some sort of buzzing sound anyway.

The picture clears from the mirror again and J, who had been sitting up under the yellow quilt watching the play of colours and the pattern of sounds, sees only the stare of his own eyes in the room. He opens a book and begins to read.

Mole sits watching J where he sits on the bed. She looks away and writes in her book, 'perhaps he is not real, does not exist, if I look up suddenly and catch him unawares he may not remember to be there.'

The room is buzzing faintly. Annie cannot discover

the source of the noise, though she moves all the objects on the kitchen table several times... The cat, orange coloured and small, comes into the room and climbs onto Mole. Annie says that the cat is like a demon. Mole reflected that Annie had said J was a demon. "But then", says Annie, "J is like a cat". Mole thought that Annie was unhappy... A coldness seemed to rise from the floor, a supernatural chill and a feeling of presence in the next room disturbed her – it was time to leave.

J feels cold in the room, so he crosses to the heap of clothes and pulls on a jacket; then he sits down, lighting a cigarette before picking a book up from the floor.

And sometimes, well sometimes Mole couldn't help thinking, couldn't help thinking about J performing in bed with Annie and Sylv. He did, didn't he? Annie must be good in bed, she talked about it anyway, and Sylv was slim and boyish so of course he'd like that.

He'd like that… She had dreamed he was a baby girl lying in a crib in a flush pink room and, taken from the cradle, he grew into a beautiful woman – not a man – too pretty and too gentle for a man, and wept too easily…

J eats a meal in his room, as it's growing dark he lights a candle. Don't look in the mirror tonight, time to go to sleep, think of Mother and blow out the candle. He blows out the candle in a long breath and turns to the wall, his back to the mirror. J is in the room, but the room has changed, there are long, glassy fissures in the mirror. The mirror is cracking, fragmenting, and the room with its objects shatters. There is a sigh, three figures ghost the room and are gone. The room and J are crumbling into dust – dissolving.

The room is empty, J is no longer reflected in the mirror – only the room looks at the room blankly.

MAUREEN OLIVER

Just One of the Family

My formative years were, perhaps, somewhat bizarre. I was a difficult child. I remember myself snarling and lurking in corners, snapping and growling at any approach. Then, of course, there were my sisters... one wore great, heavy metal studded boots and would lash out without warning to land a savage kick on shins, ankles – and, when she grew a little, any other protrusion it took her fancy to adorn with a colourful bruise. Kicker's approach would cause me to retreat further into my corner and show my teeth. Once I caught hold of her leg and ripped it, tasting blood with satisfaction and watching her great shoes make tracks for the kitchen as she let out fearful howls.

Not to forget the other dear sister, the quiet one – Sinister – who slipped noiselessly from room to room – a thin shade of a girl. Her long, pale moon face would slide out of the darkness and into my corner, the slash that served for a mouth would move and a soft hiss of barely audible expletives would drip from it. She, with her quiet evil, held me rigid with fear, for against her there could be no defence; no violence on my part could stop up that flow of malice. Long after her face had disappeared back into the darkness, a faint buzz of hatred would palpitate in the empty space. So, my youth was not jolly or carefree, and oh, then there were my parents...

My dear Mother, always doing something in the kitchen, always doing it in the kitchen while wearing Father's overcoat and a pair of carpet slippers with holes in them – yes, she was always doing it in the kitchen, although what it was she was doing exactly was a mystery, since nothing ever actually got done. She hummed cheerfully as she did it, she hummed 'bizzy, bizzy, bizzy' – she was always very busy, she was so busy she never had time to take out the combs and curlers knotted in her great pile of tangled, dusty grey hair

– she was so busy she could not stop to clean her face of the smuts that flew upon her from every corner of the smut stained room. Her fingers delved and twisted in this pile of indescribable something and then in that heap of decaying mire – whether those were the boiling socks or the evening meal I could never be quite sure.

Oh Mother, was she content back then? Was she happy in the crumbling kitchen among the dearly remembered heaps of whatever it was that littered the room lovingly? If you scratched at the grimy flooring with a little wooden stick, you might see tiny red flowers and hearts that had been covered up and hidden for many, many years. Dearest Mother, perhaps if I had scraped away the dust I would have found beautiful patterns in her too. But I would never have dared to move too close, for a swift movement of the hand, too sudden to anticipate, and I could find myself flying to a crash landing against the wall.

And Father, I remembered Father by the slam of the door and a low rumbling sound, though whether this was actually his voice or some digestive problem I cannot be sure. Father, like my younger sister, was very ready with his feet and it was advisable to steer well clear of those heavy, brown shoes. Father was not exactly unkind – often he'd risk being scarred by snapping jaws while gently tapping my head with his fist as he passed my corner, it was Father who would slide the tray of grey meat across the floor towards me – I preferred to dine alone. Though the rumbling, and those shoes, I did not altogether trust Father. Why did I go back there?

Well, after a few years I started to think that it couldn't have been quite that bad – or could it? So, I got the idea to go back just to check up. I think I had started to doubt that the Family really existed... After all, the friends I had acquired since were all gentle smiling people, beautiful people, who glided about the city as quiet as cats in great purring automobiles. The life I now lived cast doubt on the reality of my past and, after all, I had been so young when I made the break – a mere cub... Perhaps my memory was playing tricks and the shadows in my mind were just that, shadows without foundation or substance. If that were so I must know the truth, besides I needed a family, my story of being the disinherited son of a Cornish Lord was wearing a little thin. I might want to write an autobiography or something...

As I said, as a mere pup I had escaped the family home and run wild and free until I was apprehended and found myself in a corrective institution for young offenders. Here my education began, I learned the crafts of lying, of how to destroy an opponent with a smile, how to stamp on the toes of adversaries and convert them to sickening obeisance. Here I forged the ladder that would lead me on to 'make it' in the great, wonderful world of opportunity in the outside world. I was intelligent enough to make sure that my particular form of corruption would not take such a simple form as to have me imprisoned again. My manoeuvres were devious and my assaults were made with blithely smiling expressions of innocence. I knew how to destroy with gentleness, to cheat in a way that made me loved and respected by all who knew me... Three years after leaving the institution I was a success. The future seemed rosy – so why did I go back?

The door opened very slowly, and into the split of darkness slipped a pale, thin face. My heart bounced in my chest, I was poised for flight when the thin lips cracked the face in a grimace intended to be a smile. I froze in horrified fascination, and, in that moment of indecision, I was seized by those skeletal hands and pulled inside the house. The smell was choking, a kind of thick, musty cloud served as air, it was in that fetid atmosphere that I had been bred. I felt a low growl start up from my trembling guts, I could not flee, my sister held me fast. She began to call - a thin, high scream. Heavy shoes banged on the stairs and Kicker lurched towards me – her intention obvious. But her kick froze in mid-air at the sight of the cruel white mask of her sister's face. An age, and we stood confronting each other, not moving or speaking. My sisters seemed not to have grown older, but in some strange way to have, well, decayed.

Why had I come? The kitchen door opened and the full force of a blast of some stinking steam from a bubbling pot on the stove hit me. I nearly fainted but Sinister held me upright in a strong, hard grip. Mother's voice was a gentle whine of greeting. She released me from my sister and pulled me into the kitchen. I seemed to be welcome. I sat down and a cup of hot, grey liquid was set in front of me. Kicker banged down a plate of sliced meat, blood still trickling from the swollen flesh. I almost gagged.

Father had been standing behind me, slowly I

became aware of a low grumbling sound, then my neck was gripped savagely, and, as the growl in my stomach rose to a strangled howl of protest, I felt something cold grip my neck and heard the snap of a fastened clip. I was collared, I was chained, "He's grown," rumbled Father, "hurry, chain him to something." Briefly, they all paused to stare around the room for a suitable object. I took my chance. I bit deep into Father's hand, and, as he released his grip on the leash, I raced from the room and out of the house, the heavy steel chain flapping at my back: I was young and strong – I outwitted them and escaped.

For a few days I hid out in an empty warehouse by the docks, stealing food from the dustbins of nearby houses at night, slinking around walls and behind corners, fearful of being seen, conscious of the chain still about my neck that, struggle as I might, I could not unfasten. After a while, however, I reasoned that the Family knew nothing of my recent comfortable existence and, hiding the chain as best I could, I returned, under cover of darkness, to my apartment on the other side of town.

It was some little time before I could summon the courage to leave that sanctuary – but at last I returned to my business, under the pretext of having been taken suddenly ill. There I was afforded due consideration – kind words were expressed as to my having made a full recovery. Yet, was it my imagination or did I receive strange, sidelong glances? My assistants kept their distance and seemed afraid that I might inadvertently touch them or brush against them. I fancied I heard anxious whispering behind my back, and, when I came into a room, conversation would cease and an unnatural silence would ensue. Perhaps it was the chain, which, try as I might, I could not remove. My attempts to disguise it had been so feeble that I had taken to letting it swing free hoping it might be thought a fashion statement – in the past I had been seen as something of a trendsetter... I began to see, however, that I was now regarded as an eccentric, and perhaps a dangerous eccentric at that...

I was at a party given by someone who had once been a close friend. My associates, however, had invited me this time, since they were too afraid to deny me the pleasure. Pleasure it was not, in fact, and I stood alone drinking in a corner, brooding on my recent misfortunes and eyeing the gambolling of my former friends with a cynical eye. As I turned away to get another drink, I sensed a hush fall upon the room and heard a muffled scream. I looked around into the grinning mask-like face of Sinister. In a flash, Father had seized the chain, Kicker was doing her best to break my shin bone with her steel-capped boots and Mother held me tight in a sooty paw. I yelled to my companions for help but they stood still, making no attempt to come to my aid. Helplessly I thrashed about, snapping and tearing at my Father. A partygoer ran forward, I thought he was coming to help me, but he stripped off his tie and bound my jaws together. As I was dragged away, I heard a great sigh of relief go up from the assembled group, then whispering, giggling – laughter.

After that, I ceased to struggle and allowed myself to be led through the dark streets. It was raining. I remember that the cool rain comforted me and drove the burning tears away from my eyes.

I am almost happy now. Sometimes they release me from my chains and allow me to run around the locked yard. I belong here – I am, after all, just one of the Family.

House

See black, see dark, see shaft of light illumine softening angle of face flowing into the night, see puddle of eyes open, see cavern of mouth open. The words shaping in her head stopped the sound bubbling in her throat, and she threw off the covers and old coats that were keeping her warm, where she lay in the smell and the dark.

Oh, turn the light on, oh, wrap the darling ripeness of body's pink and sweat and turn to face the room. The bulb reflecting the mirror burned with a fierce yellow that cut the eyes, but pacing a few steps into the quiet and it was a white face and staring eyes that looked out from under the tangle of greying hair and gaped at itself. Mirror taking my face, she thought, mirror eating my soul, mirror that took me young and laughing, mirror that waits for me old and dying – oh...

She found a cigarette on the floor and sat down mid the clothes and empty tins and thought, time to think, and thought, but it seemed something watched - laughing - in the corner. It was only a girl, but she wished it would go away. It would not be so happy if it knew its fate was here - its fate? But something else waited behind her, she could not make it out, but - oh... The smell of it was decaying and she dared not turn around. Better leave it to its gentle rotting.

She found a dragon shaped ink stain on the carpet that seemed strangely portentous but could not think for why. A dragon lying upon a rock, sunning itself gently – beneath the thick crust of corroded green the soft flesh throbbed intensely, the rhythm of the ice blood slipped slime around the cold bones.

The gas fire burning reflected in the mirror, and a young girl, naked, waiting expectantly curled up on a narrow bed, feeling, 'I won't be able to, there's sure to be something wrong with me, some deformity of mind and body, not like other women.' And the toothpaste smiles on the television...then he was a virgin too...

How long had she been in the room? The laughing girl peering in at the mirror now; she did not live in the room, but the wild face with the dream encircled eyes did, and she could not face the shades of decay that lay in the darkest shadowed corner – the corner of the room she dared not face. Those shades had lain in the room for all time, and other shades: some smiling, some crying, some heated in passion, some old in prayer – worn knees on the mat before the clouded window - filled the room. Yet she was all that was in the room. A young woman in the mirror, fear in her eyes.

The house by the canal stood alone, the other houses demolished, the street white and deserted in the October sunlight. I moved in. The house smelled rather musty. I opened all the windows and saw a swan float by. Later, I ate lemon cake and wished I had a radio, some noise to fight the blackness of the empty starless sky that stared in at me. I heard scuffling on the stairs that might have been rats. Slept, and dreamed fitfully of purple faces and laughter, awoke cold, the windows were all still open.

Somehow it didn't seem to matter any more - the washing and the clothes changing. There was little future, only nightmares and half-remembered dreams from future or past. I wished the shadows wouldn't clump together and stare accusingly at me. Shadows coloured purple slid green-eyed in the dark. Days and nights became confused – sometimes I slept through the day, sometimes the night, or perhaps day and night – I could not tell. Sometimes I went out to walk aimlessly. I spoke to no one and no one spoke to me. Figures were beginning to appear indistinct and the grey web faces I saw were dissolving into the substance of the walls of the house. People became the mere sound of steady, insistent breathing, sometimes close by, sometimes faint and distant, but when I looked for them all I saw were faint shapes, the occasional bone and skin, fingers, and still watching eyes.

I went out less and less often. Somehow the house seemed to have acquired a personality. It needed me. Shadows on the walls formed amorphous faces watching calmly, yet threatening and disturbing. Then the walls seemed to breathe with me. Rhythmically, steadily they pulsed, inhaled, exhaled with a slight hissing sound. The colour of the walls would change subtly, sometimes beautifully – green to purple to aquamarine to deep blue and purple again.

One night, eating chips and feeling clear in the head but oppressed by solitude, I thought I'd visit the local pub where college students gathered. I might find a friend, someone would speak to me –

maybe someone I knew.

A cheerful group, drinks at the table. I sat down and they smiled, all welcoming eyes. I smiled too. I answered questions. Loud music drowned conversation. A warm leg nudged mine. He walked home with me. I was pleased because the streets down to the canal were dark and I was afraid. I liked him – he held my arm. Then he pushed his way into the house asking for coffee. I was surprised to find the walls were red. He tripped over a pile of dirty clothes on the floor and I smiled politely. He was big and dark, with nearly black eyes, and I liked his tip-tilted mouth and the way his eyes creased when he smiled. Then he grabbed at me and the touch of his fingers burnt my skin. The house darkened. I resisted the claw of his fingers with a regretful smile. His hands insisted and tore at my dress. The walls became black and the house simmered with protest at the invasion. The man animal filled my vision. I raged at his demanding greed – his face was a mask, his eyes black puddles. Trousers round his knees he fell toward me; arms stretched out, the giant purple prick comic in its despair. I pushed him and he fell against the door, bruising his head and gashing his cheek – the sight of his blood filled me with satisfying thoughts of hacking him into a messy heap and I remembered a sharp knife in the kitchen and fetched it. I brandished it at his genitals and he gathered up his pants and fled into the night. I laughed, and then felt weak. The walls pulsed purple again and beat like a great heart pounding, desperate to stay alive in a weakening body. The house disapproved of copulation. I slept for a long time.

Days and nights passed. Over the house I felt the silence of the stars in the blanket of sky. The walls shone and pulsed, and in the grope of darkness shapes were formed and shadowy figures moved and breathed.

The wild face reflected in the still eye of the mirror.

The woman sat down heavily on the bed, her mouth opening and closing – fish-like amaze in the pale of her face. Shadows moved about the room, darkened the mirror and moved on. Delicate sounds, like the soft humming of bees on a summer's day in a rose garden, filled the air. She lay down, stuffing her face with a ragged sheet and covered her body with an old coat of animal fur. She lay there for some time while the humming intensified and words became distinguishable here and there in the well of sound.

She awoke; the moaning in the room was getting louder. Brain aching in striated web of pain. Body crumpled weak, face green, glazed - granny smith apple pale, and eyes searching the blinding dark seeing only mind pictures. Jewelled peacock eye's centre, coloured wheels of light spitting fire. Whirls blazing life to the departing, hands stilled, claws clutched at soiled bed sheets. Dank smell. The room shadowed with figures shaping the gloom, reflecting averted eyes in the mirror's stare.

Pictures, more pictures: laughing child, mother knitting by a blaze of fire glow, light coruscating around the curled shape of her head, warm circled – umbilical union – faces flowing in the water, faces merging with other faces – dreaming; the quiet room. Pinched finger ends arranging flowers in a jam jar. Thinking 'I am growing old here', yet there is a strange pleasure in the resignation as the mirror catches the brilliant colours of anemones in a flood. Darkening eyes – must see, must see – don't put the light out Mummy please, don't Mummy, it's dark, Mummy please...

Pain ceasing, cold spreading from feet to head, eyes want to close. '*I not gone*'. Dark walls crushing me and I see my face – my faces – grouped together in the mirror that stares through its eye at this *I*. Heads turn away – don't go – oh, the dark, no shape, no colour, no smell, no feel, no pain, no sense, no nothing any more.

The young woman entered the rented house by the canal and opened all the windows wide. 'This will do fine', she thought. Then she noticed a dragon shaped inkblot on the carpet and it made her shudder slightly. Shaking off the feeling and smiling, she looked up and saw herself darkly reflected in a mirror....

Room

This, then, is my all. This is my room, my life; there could be nothing before this. There is no future but this. This is a rectangle of silver-grey vibrant material, light, constantly refreshing the eyes with rainbows of reflected colour. Within it I dwell upon my bed – my large, soft bed, covered with satin smooth sheets, which slide comforting, cool, over my warm flesh. I dwell within the boundaries of this flesh, soft pink flesh on soft pink sheets in a gentle world of pastel colours. Colours seemingly reflected from a square of window that I cannot reach. My only pain is the provoking needle of curiosity. Why the window? Agonies of speculation – what can be beyond the comfort of Room? A possibility of endless rooms progressing to infinity stretches my imagination to a degree that threatens the equilibrium of mind.

I cannot reach the window. Even if there was some object to stand on, the bed is riveted to the floor and the chains attached to the manacles around my wrists are too short. I cannot even reach the windowed wall. I can see a square of constantly changing light – the light of a vast otherness – of a room that encloses all rooms.

The Servicer comes, a white faced silence, empty eyed it feeds me with pleasurable substances, checks my body heat controls, adjusts the flow of soothing sounds... The Servicer does, but thinks not. Behind the empty eyes: more emptiness, vacancy. Controlled by...I know not...is there control? There must be control, there must be a system that organizes Servicers, that produces the pleasurable sensations that surround me, a control that has provided the pain, the freedom to speculate, afforded by the existence of the window. If there is a Controller, why did it lance the comfort of this life with the pain of unknowing? If it weren't for the window there would be simplicity, security. For what reason does the window exist? Unknowing burns me. I direct my gaze at the flowing colours upon the glowing wall opposite. I am absorbed in the seductive pleasure afforded by the exact and complex harmonies of hue. Discomfort subsides to a vague awareness, my mind is one with the room; colours and sounds thrill my body.

The Servicer has removed the manacles and is massaging my wrists with smooth, firm strokes of its cool metallic fingers. Colours intensify, purples and greens flood the optic nerve, fill the brain with soporific sweetness, I am almost overcome by the desire to sleep, sinking into an ultramarine sea of unconsciousness...

Discordant sounds, loud and unpleasant; violent reds suffuse the walls. The Servicer emits a shrill, loud sound. It sways and tumbles to the ground, still buzzing faintly and, from the walls, instead of delicate music and fine colours – horrible groaning, moaning sounds, crashes and roars, the walls change from red to black. I can move, I can get up, I must feel my way in this darkness to the window – I must reach the window. The effort of standing causes considerable discomfort, but I do stand. I move cautiously. Save for the dull pink light from the window, all is darkness, is quiet but for a hiss, a crackle, a very faint moan from beyond the wall. The window is above me, just out of my reach – I cannot reach the window.

I crouch in the darkness. I cannot reach the window. Flesh tinted light glows pale on the metal body of the Servicer rendering the now disarrayed limbs to the semblance of a mutilated human body. The Servicer...its metal body will allow me to reach the window! I drag the heavy torso across the room. Conscious of choking fumes I am having difficulty breathing. It has become almost hot enough to sear the flesh form the bones. I snatch the, now useless, hand of the Servicer from a tangle of wires and climb upon its torso...

I can see through the window! I can see! I can

see! But there is nothing – save indistinct shapes – there are no walls! Fearfully I raise the metal hand and the window is broken. I climb out, I bleed, but I am free! Free is a space without walls. But there must be walls. I cannot conceive of a space without walls...when the mist clears I shall see them. This outer room is large indeed – but what a foolish thought it was to even dream of a space without walls...

Red light fills the space, looking up I can hardly see the ceiling of this strangeness, this vast outer room. Behind me the building is consumed in red. I move rapidly away from the heat and the smoke. Now I can see. The walls, where are the walls? I cannot live in a space without walls. Colours litter the place untidily – without pattern, without plan. Fear grips me and I cannot move. This is the abomination I was shielded from, this was what was outside the window: boundless chaos... space without order, desolation. I fall to the ground. I feel – hunger, cold, the ache of fear. Here I will die – I

am already dying – for Room is no more and there
is no window to reach.

MAUREEN OLIVER

Poetry

Lilacs and Other Flowers

All the psyche wards have names of

Flowers

As if some sweet

Scent

Could disguise the odour of

Decay.

So with deepest

Dread

I hear the word:

Lilacs

And a death bell

Tolls

'Abandon hope all ye who enter –

Here'.

At least isolation has its

Pleasures,

Moving from bed to

Sofa,

Switching on the TV, the

Radio,

Crying along to an old

Song,

Or just talking

Back to the thin, yet densely peopled

Air.

To be alone is far better than

Being

Just another

Hybrid

In the garden of lost

Souls.

2004

The Conversation

The air hangs in folds of ice between
us,
Something touches my cheek –
So cold, so cold;
My body burns, strangled with
impotent emotion.

The flow of thought splinters, diverts;
I hear the ice
Melt, dripping into the silence.
Language struggles to unite us,
You are closer, close, but
No, a deft turn of phrase and the
fragile
Bond is severed.

An abstruse chill, snow crystals
pattern
The space between us.

MAUREEN OLIVER

Your hair is haloed silver,
Cool against the sunlit window.

1978

When We First Met

We were together,

I dug my fingers into the pocket

Of your rough tweed coat.

It was very cold,

Not quite winter,

I crunched dry leaves with my heels,

And we laughed at our breath

Ice bound in the still air.

1976

Doctor's Orders

"You're getting old, dear lady,"
The doctor said,
"And your skin has become very pale,
It's really quite white, and my dear, it's not right
For your eyes to be black circled so.
I suggest my dear, for your health, it's quite clear,
Some routine life you must follow.
Give up on daydreaming on nighttimes spent scheming –
Those plans from which no fruits show.
Can't you see it's all vanity?
T'will lead to insanity.
Reject agitation,
Take up vegetation,
Start a graceful decline,

Your age says it's time,

Stop twisting and turning,

Your brains they are burning.

Don't weave fantasies at night

They just give you a fright,

Take up knitting and crochet –

Now listen to what I say,

My advice you must take,

For the sake of your future

Stop messing with culture

It really don't suit yer,

As I said, you grow older,

Don't be bolder –

Be colder

My dear."

1979

Boy Blue

Little Boy Blue,

Sighs and shining eyes,

Stirring coffee and pining –

'Oh secret sadness, oh tragedy,'

Could I help him? Oh motherly me.

"Let me talk to you, so sweet and kind,

So helpful, so nice, let me show you my mind."

Oh charming, oh sad, emotionally pure,

You might think him sensitive,

You may well be wrong.

Oh, motherly ladies from Whitby to Poole

Are waiting the visit of Little Boy Blue.

The ladies who understand sad little boys

Are wanting to comfort him, offer him toys.

SHORT STORIES & POETRY

You might think him an angel,

You may be deluded.

The ladies who offered this cherub their all

Are lying to husbands, some in the grave,

Some knotted in strait jackets –

But the comfort they gave!

Some have taken to drink, some in therapy,

Some gave him their money,

Some just offered tea.

Oh kindly ladies from Whitby to Poole

Don't give him sweeties; don't warm him in bed,

Don't talk with him; offer him spiritual aid.

Your heart will be emptied; your soul will be raped

For he swallows them whole, he digests them all,

Those kind helpful ladies, from Whitby to Poole.

1978

Trust

Trust, they tell me

is what I need.

"Trust me, trust us and

we will pour oil on those

wounds, we will heal your pain,

if you only trust in us."

The mask seems golden,

the smile benign,

light plays around the hollows

of the eyes,

russet shadows flicker lovingly

across cheekbones, and

I am enticed, almost under a spell.

Faltering, trusting, I reveal my secrets,

like some damned dance of the Seven Veils

in Hell, till, vulnerable in my innocence

I observe with horror that

dark lies and rude cruelty now

stain the welcoming visage, and,

at the portal of Hades, I hesitate,

turn back to retrace my steps, but

flight is impossible for

he holds the seeds

of my soul in his palm – and

now winningly,

the therapist smiles –

showing his teeth.

2006

At Seventeen

Seventeen she was, the girl

living alone in that house,

the empty ruin by the canal.

She met a man, older than she,

they had a drink, or two or three.

It grew late; the way back was long and dark –

scary.

The man seemed friendly,

said he'd see her safely home.

They reached her door,

she said goodnight,

then he grabbed her, and, as

the house swallowed them up,

he tore at her, ripping

at her clothes, her hair, her skin.

SHORT STORIES & POETRY

It seemed the walls went purple

and red shadows danced about the room.

She yelled, nobody heard – poor cow!

Didn't she know only a slut, a tart,

would let him walk her home

that way? She did not.

He was getting nowhere

so he changed his tactics

and brought her to her knees.

So much pain and fear, disgust

and shame for her to bear –

but it was the humiliation

she would remember

all her living days, in that room

with the purple shadows

and the demons dancing red upon the walls

in the empty house, where, later, he left her

alone – except for the rats.

2006

Hands

You say softly,

'My hands are growing old'.

You turn and turn them,

Extending fingertips,

Examining palms,

With uneasy alarm.

My hands I do not care to

Examine; claw fisted,

Thrust into pockets.

1978

MAUREEN OLIVER

The Misunderstanding

If there were some bridge I could

Meet you on,

Some space between two spaces,

Crossing water,

Surrounded by mist.

Then I could tell you,

And you could tell me.

1977

Just Like Jimmy Stewart

Just like Jimmy Stewart

in some old black and white movie

I have always yearned,

always reached out for

that elusive, shimmering dream.

Just like him, I want to

lasso the moon.

2004

At the High Table

Sitting in a wine bar

at a great, high table,

from where I survey

the babbling, bibbing

rabble below,

I remember schooldays –

how my headmistress also

sat raised upon a platform above us

at meal times.

She'd glower down at

the mucky, gym slipped girls,

her gimlet eyes sharpened to observe

the flying brussel sprout,

the upturned bowl of sago pudding,

or perhaps a screeching child

ripe for punishment.

She was always alert, ready

to forestall any frolic

that might disturb the dignity,

the peace, of that shared repast –

our school dinner.

But here its wine not water

that we drink, and I fancy myself a

benevolent overseer

observing the lads and lasses busily

flirting, drinking, feeding, and yes

screeching too…

Still, just like my old headmistress

I sit alone and try, unsuccessfully,

to eat my food – with grace.

2005

According to Sharon

Two Catholic matrons –

Sharon and me

sit over tea,

discussing the late

great Pope,

Church affairs, and

the problems of being single

mothers who try

to stay

faithful and pure.

Words flow, and

we find warmth

in our common ground.

We witness our faith

while smoking and laughing

in a Wimbledon café.

Then the conversation

turns to dissenters,

feminists clashing with

the Old Ways of

our beloved, patriarchal,

yet *Mother* Church.

We touch on what some call

'Reproductive Rights',

nodding sagely in agreement, saying,

'that is *wrong,* this is *right* –

according to Tradition,

to Revealed Truth.'

Then she tells me, casually,

"Women must be prepared

to die, if need be. So that

the unborn child, still in the

womb, might survive."

She says it's mandatory

for Catholic women

and my eyes widen

in shocked disbelief.

She says she would have given up

her own life

without a qualm

so that her sons

might survive birth – and her.

Feeling inadequate

I cannot frame the words 'me too'.

I am in awe –

is she *so* much better than me?

Afterward, I remember –

she has no daughters,

no little girl like my

grandchild,

who, when she smiles

or frowns

pictures my mother's look –

a woman she can never meet

in this life.

Sharon has no daughters,

no granddaughters, to cause

icy fear to freeze her soul

as it does mine,

at the thought of such

a bloody, female sacrifice.

2005

Burning the Book

We sat together by the blazing

coal fire that night

just as any other.

By the fire where we used to

toast bread on forks,

till the forks grew so hot

we'd burn our fingers

and laugh.

So we sat there, and

big brother produced

his philosophical stance,

his atheism,

persuasive, logical;

while I cradled my fat, black Book,

bound in gold, against my chest and

rocked and wept,

crying, "No, no, no."

Finally, he seemed to win, and,

as proof, exhorted me to throw

the Bible into the flames.

I did so, expecting a thunderbolt –

waited to be struck dead,

but it was only Mum

standing in the doorway, calling us both

"Wicked".

Yet I did lose my faith that night –

I lost my belief in the absolute infallibility of

my wonderful, big brother.

2005

The Lost Boy

I saw him again

yesterday, the Lost Boy,

still in that same baby blue

school sweatshirt.

This Catholic child with the face of

an angel,

an angel unaccountably fallen –

fallen here among us.

We are mere shades in our own

personal Hell –

a demon on each one's shoulder.

About the once shining youth there is still

a detectable, faintly shimmering, radiance,

hope's innocent halo –

but tarnished, fading now.

Today his hair is two-tone,

one side bright bleach yellow.

He cracks a joke. "It was a bargain, I got it done

half-price". Then he lights a cigarette,

twisting his mouth into a crooked grin –

and everyone smiles.

2006

You and the Tarot

_Woman, you are Knight of Swords,

Do you attack or defend my castle walls?

Your essence shimmers, overflows,

Ignites, and falls burning to the ground.

I sense your pain – but I am afraid of pain,

Toil, tears, grief...

I am Queen of Cups,

The lazy, meandering river's flow,

The dark side of the moon, the Hermit,

The gentle witch.

My several persons are sundered

By the passion, the rage in you.

You are a red rose in full flower –

With needle sharp thorns.

1986

The Angel and Emily Aged Three

Dreams, messages,

Emily saw a man in the tree,

He was polishing his wings, said she

Just before dinner –

But I saw nothing,

Only drew the blinds

And ate in silence.

1973

MAUREEN OLIVER

Visiting Verulaneum

The high wall – indigo shadowed, rust rimmed –

Is now topped with grass,

Children playing on it,

Dandelions cluttered under it.

Green, and splashes of yellow,

With emerald clumps on the purple –

Stone is cold.

Here in the rubble filled spaces, people once

Lived; eating, drinking and

Finally dying under skies like this

Our blue one.

Today the clouds move thinly over the latticed,

Tree spangled countryside.

Boys climb the old city walls

And there are lolly sticks in the underground

shrine.

The bones of dead Sixtus –

'Died aged about twenty – male'

Are composed tidily in the small museum.

Scraps of bone and hair, teeth and fingernails, rest

Quietly under the soil.

Visitors wheeling pushchairs

Retire to suppers and secret affairs.

The gates are locked,

The museum is closed,

Sixtus still sleeps.

Venus steps out of her shrine,

Delicately, over crumpled coke cans,

Amid the detritus of the living.

1972

MAUREEN OLIVER

Woman to Woman

Like the delicate dripping

of water between stalactite and

stalagmite, slowly, steadily

seeps my love

for you.

Like a great river

meandering between

fields of yellow and green,

softly, gently flows my love

for you.

My love is firm like the oak

soaring heavenward,

brilliant like the heat of the summer sun,

enduring as a rock standing firm

against the constant onslaught of the

restless sea.

Delicate, fragile as a moonbeam and

strong as a tiger –

ferociously, tenderly

my love

enfolds you.

In the twin echoes of

our beating hearts

moment flows into moment –

ecstatic union of souls,

our breathing conjoined –

softly, silently I have given myself to you,

as we lie embracing –

haloed by the pure gold of our passion.

1995

Light in Darkness

Filled with a new and raw

grief,

I scurried through the rain-soaked

greyness

of the hospital grounds –

to a solitary bench

to shelter.

I lit a cigarette,

alone with my anguish.

Very soon, I had two companions –

a tired and worn elderly man

and a young black woman,

her head covered in a

brightly coloured scarf.

We three sat together

and smoked and talked,

and talked and talked.

"My brother has only a short time

To live", I said

in answer to their questions.

Then I heard how she had sickle cell

and her life was a constant round

of hospital visits and pain,

and how he too was under sentence,

departing this world slowly –

bit by precious bit.

Watching the ambulances come and go

in the driving rain,

I listened and noted

her lively mind

and his resilience.

Very soon, we were smiling,

telling stories –

laughing, and I sensed the beating

of wings, for the

Angel of Comfort was

close by.

In the greyness

of twilight,

for a little while,

the dim evening was

suffused with colour –

and life.

2002

MAUREEN OLIVER

Prescription

They tell me I am too, too happy, or
too, too sad.
Oh, altogether too much –
absolutely *mad.*
"Take this pill", they say,
"and this,
you'll be calm and quiet,
still and sane,
watch TV
and sleep all night,
then come and see us –
we'll make you right".

I tried the pills,
they made me sleep
not just at night –
no time to weep –
no time to laugh –
no time to sing –
slowly, slowly

vegetating.

Sleep till midday,
eat
and sleep some more.
no energy,
no hope, no future,
no art, no culture –
no total despair –
just boredom; ennui,
no sudden leap
of joy,
no spirituality.

Sod the pills,
precious life slips by
so surely,
I want to taste it
dregs and all,
I want to feel it
in all its tattered glory.

Take back your pills,
its courage we need
on this journey
and the vital spark,
the living breath –
inspiration –
not living death.

2003

Sister

'She is like your sister', he observed with a smile.

She is like my sister,

Her thought is like clouds ravelling, unravelling,

Her skies changing swiftly,

Storms in an instant,

Spears in those fierce eyes.

Her night cloaked soul flies about her

Woolly, wild head,

Her dreams crown a hawk's skull

With nightmare.

As she talks, her small hands weave

Circles in inner space.

But she is like my sister,

I can almost reach the clouds.

Smoking endless cigarettes,

Blowing out smoke,

Those clouds pass behind her eyes.

Yes, she is like my sister –

But the weather changes,

And then I fear the gaze of the hawk.

1977

Babylon Woman

Shuffling through

the streets of this

Babylon

with the help

of my trusty cane,

I think of you, and you,

and you.

Your faces swim bleakly

through my memory –

palely, mocking me.

And now again

I hear the voices,

acerbic, cruel.

My fingers bled

from holding on too tight,

so I let go

and fell,

breaking everything –

breaking down.

2004

After the Silent Running

After the silent running,

going nowhere fast,

eyes stung by uncried tears,

holding on to her pain

and smiling,

she wanted her friends to love her…

too much.

She wanted –

a hug, a cup of strong, sweet tea,

a voice saying, 'It'll be alright,

I care.'

But it was not to be,

sensing she was other than she

they withdrew.

Doors closed in her face,

no one called for a chat

anymore.

Alone but for her cat,

within the nailed down box of

four walls,

surrounded by the ruins of

her life,

she wept.

2004

Detritus

Clear away the debris,

detritus scattered

by lost and lonely angels,

piled thickly, silver

and grey and white, and find

flecked, blackened wires of –

is it hair?

Search, dig deep, and

there you may

uncover a mask,

a face, perhaps

twisted into a smile

or grimace.

Joy, pain –

pleasure?

Only Heaven knows –

or Hell maybe…

2006

You Can't Cuddle a God

It's all very well consorting

With gods and goddesses,

Radiant in glory – ineffable,

Coruscating hallowed holy divinity –

Omnipotent deities.

It's all very well conversing

With a carved and perfect

Face of stone,

Or sensing the Mother Goddess

Thrill in the earth,

It's all very well but…

If you reach out in the dark night

To touch them

There's only empty air there.

MAUREEN OLIVER

Well might your arms ache…

You can't cuddle a god.

1984

What Do You Want?

What do you want of me woman?

I am a tired old moggie cat,

I walk alone,

My eyes are green,

I've seen things you have never seen,

One of my legs is wonky

And my back hurts,

Yet, I still hunt alone.

It'd be good to curl up and cuddle with you

Against the dark night,

But always I have one foot on the ground

Ready for flight.

I don't want to hurt you,

I care for you

In my way,

But I am a tired old moggie cat

And I hunt alone.

I'll stay with you,

Sleep on your mat,

Sit by your fire,

Rub my dark head on your bosom,

But always I must be free to go –

Cats are wild

They cannot be owned.

1986

Normal

You give me drugs to make me

normal.

You say I have some illness that

has taken normality

away from me –

I tell you now, I never was, nor could be

normal.

At school they knew me for what I was

and would have none of me,

they made it clear they knew I was not

normal.

Therapy was tried and failed, and

drugs made me stupid, but, lamentably, still not

normal.

MAUREEN OLIVER

Leave me alone! I am not normal!

I was never meant to be –

give me my books and my paintings,

let me listen to the Magic Flute,

let me talk to myself,

let me dream

awake

till I die, and afterwards let my epitaph be –

'Sadly, the trouble with her was

she was never really quite

normal'.

2005

The Nutter on the Bus

I am that celebrated

nutter on the bus,

clutching my pass I

climb aboard.

Midst nervous coughs and

shuffling feet

I seat myself next to

a grey-haired woman with

a kindly face,

and start to chat

'bout weather and stuff.

But she shifts awkwardly, and

nervously submits

the misty rain spattered window

pane to an alarmed

stare.

I must be that famous nutter because

now I am mumbling under my breath.

Just another trick of the senses –

I merely thought someone wanted

to speak to me.

Sometimes, I forget

I am just

that celebrated, almost famous

nutter on the bus.

2005

The Rainbow

When I was little, I looked up and saw

God's covenant in the sky –

the rainbow.

I counted all her brilliant colours and knew

that in some hidden place

was a cache of purest gold,

the treasure of my dreams

come to fruition.

I grew up searching,

searching for that vision,

'Where your treasure is

there will your heart be also'.

My song was, 'Somewhere over the Rainbow',

I sang it through my childhood –

as I sing it still.

Maturity brought some sorrow,

but, still I look for that

Rainbow's-End.

Growing old, I am battered from

the Quest, from fighting to attain

the Grail of a child's hope;

yet still I seek, and in that seeking

I live.

2004

To You

One evening, a cool evening in late summer,

as I sat in my garden

in the gathering dark –

the sky had grown stormy,

redolent of unshed rain,

I looked up and saw swarms

of starlings flying overhead,

flying south,

ever south.

I saw the little black birds gathered

together

in clusters,

driven by some instinctual urge

to fly

quickly, quickly

through the gathering gloom.

And I remembered many, many years ago

when it all began –

you and I together in the

unexpected cold –

in London,

St James Park.

I was holding your hand inside your

coat against the chill evening.

Together we looked up

at the flying, fluttering hordes

above us,

flying south,

ever south.

And I felt such a consuming passion

for you,

for life,

for our future.

Now it seems just a dream.

I had fled from everything dear to me –

my Church, my God – family, friends,

a life – for you.

Down all the years, I recollected it then,

alone in my garden

in the failing light,

listening to the sounds of families

in the nearby houses,

watching a solitary cat walk the wall.

The starlings are gone to their fate,

and I shed a tear –

and remember.

2002

The Therapist's Question

I talk and talk, and she

listens dutifully as I

calculate and total

the sum of my experience.

Of being one

who has spent so many

years added up,

subtracted, taken away,

yet still without a

solution.

I speak with easy familiarity of

my friends, who,

have also been

compartmentalised,

medicated, sometimes put away –

out of sight, out of mind.

Then she says to me,

"Why, when you speak of *those* people

do you always say *we*?"

I am silenced briefly, then,

in a flash

she has come to sit beside me

on the comfortable sofa –

very close to me,

very close. And

she says, "*I* am your sister,

We are the same, you and I".

Clumsily, I touch her hand, not knowing

quite what to do or say,

what on earth does she *mean?*

Later, I remember when

MAUREEN OLIVER

Sisterhood was powerful – yet

there was no warmth,

no welcome from *those* sisters

when I emerged from the Psyche Ward shaken,

fragile – alone. Instead

doors closed in my face, but then

there were new friends; others just like me.

Yes, dear therapist, even the mad have

community.

2005

Bluebell Woods

It occurred to me

that morning, very early,

how I'd always dwelt

on the pains and unhappiness'

of childhood.

The unkind word, the slap, the hurt

that would not go away.

Then, a flood of memories from long ago

filled me with a nostalgic joy.

On weekends, when we were small,

Mum would pack sandwiches,

and take us off on train or bus

to nearby Kent,

to Chislehurst Common and Petts Wood –

the Bluebell Woods.

In spring the flowers were a carpet of blue,

we'd gather them up in armfuls.

Big brother and me running in and out of the trees;

the great oaks and the elegant willows.

'Hide and Seek' and 'Catch Me If You Can',

laughing and playing

in the bright, gentle warmth of the day.

The rhododendrons were hung with huge

blossoms,

red and purple.

You could crawl inside

flower-filled bushes

and make a secret space where

no one could see you,

curled up tight,

surrounded by the dark green leaves,

safe.

Somewhere, hidden in the forest,

was a clearing –

we always came upon it with surprise.

It felt magical that field of tufted grasses.

And there were 'fairy rings'

where the winged imps would dance –

but only when we weren't looking.

It was whispered that if you

jumped three times in the ring

you'd be grabbed by an evil witch

and dragged down deep into the horrors

of Hell – never to return.

In autumn we'd go blackberrying,

and there were caves

deep, dark and mysterious –

or so Mum said.

She never took us there

though we begged her.

She'd got lost inside once

in impenetrable blackness –

terrified,

and there were bats…

Back to the woods

for more laughter and games,

and corned beef sandwiches with fizzy lemonade.

Mum could feel free for a while too

from money worries and the washing up.

She'd laugh with us,

then hold me by the hand

all the way home.

2003

Forever Eve

Sometimes, it seems, I am forever Eve

reaching out for the apple,

waiting by the Tree of Knowledge

for that fruit to fall –

Good or Evil.

Oh, make my restless proud spirit

be still for a while.

Like a querulous child

I question, question,

making endless objections,

struggling to understand

everything.

Such foolishness –

perhaps if I could be quiet

for long enough,

I might hear the answers.

Not in rhetoric,

but in music borne on

the wings of the spirit –

in the sweet sounds of angels

singing praises.

2003

The Meal

He cooked her a meal,

Fresh trout in a dish

All plump and gleaming.

"I know they're done when

Their eyes go pop"

She was all done when

Her eyes popped –

Laid out on the bed sheet

White and gleaming.

1983

Communication

Sometimes I'd like to touch you,

Put an arm around you,

Some physical communication –

Something...

Why are we afraid of contact?

Sometimes I'd like to touch you,

Seeing you happy

Join hands and dance,

Seeing you weep

Fall down crying.

Sometimes I want to touch you...

Seeing me you retreat –

Behind a smiling mask.

1975

Winter in the Park

Here was a mist – ice held,

Figures scarce moving.

A silent winter prayer,

Communication,

Conjunction of

Matter and Spirit.

Clay deep, roots quivered,

The lake grey

Reflecting sky.

White gull movements –

The entire wild, roaring Universe held

In the palm of Heaven.

1971

Supernewhousewifewoman - Or, "Oh me? I'm just a housewife..."

I am the homemaker

The all-important egg breaker,

The child shaker

The cake baker

The pill taker

The friendly, neighbourhood

Muck raker.

I am – the essential –

The mother, the wife,

The tiny, insignificant cog

That turns the Wheel of Life.

I am the Woman,

I rise at five,

Having ascertained they're all alive –

Again.

MAUREEN OLIVER

I press their clothes,

Stir porridge,

Make tea,

Wash dishes –

Then they're gone

And I'm here –

Just me?

Oh, it's great being

The smart, the clean

Supernewhousewifewoman.

I think I'll pinch myself to

See that I'm real –

Was I asleep again?

Sometimes I feel...

Don't Panic.

1976.

For my Mother – who thinks it's about time I went

to IKEA and got some decent furniture...

If I live to be old

I shall not care

I shall wear

My white hair

Screwed into a bun

And pinned.

I shall keep four cats,

Big and sleek and fat,

Sitting on separate multicoloured mats.

I shall live in a huge, empty house

With windows that stare

And never go to IKEA

Or buy pine furniture there.

1981

Willow

The weeping willow

That wept all through

The sun and raindrop

Rainbow patterned days

Of the tear stained face

Of childhood

Cries still

In the lonely dark

After the gates close

In the park.

1977.

Passion

Density of passion thins

The structure of self,

The body fragile

As brittle glass –

Smooth, nakedly empty.

Save for the insistent saying

Over and over again,

The sweet rhythm of the beloved's name.

Observe desire

Rising in the blood sap,

The nerves tense,

The bones ache,

The kernel of being

Is drowned in otherness.

1978

Spring

The spring is full of ghosts,

Shimmering reflections in the new sun's light,

Passages of past time echo, and,

Always, just around the next corner,

Waits what was

And what could have been.

This is the true New Year

When the blood quickens again,

And this fresh spring,

So new, so expectant of the future,

Is at the same time – the past.

Ages and ages condensed in

A second of sparkling sunlight;

The daffodils are yellow –

As they always were

As they always will be

For ever and ever –

Alpha and Omega,

Amen.

1978

Ship of Fools

Together they sail

in the Ship of Fools

each one lost in secret dreams –

dreams of pleasure

and lust and power;

mad with

hope they

drift through the luminescent green

unknowing seas so

enraptured by remorseless visions

they do not notice

how their ship

is sinking.

2006.

Psychosis

She held on tightly

to her dreams

only to find herself holding just

a handful

of dust.

Desperately trying to impel

herself forward

she sped back

into endless darkness;

the tunnel sucked her in and down –

and then there was the fire.

The hissing of the flames

rang in her ears,

a whispering hollow sound –

a nightmare of demonic voices

taunting, deriding her till

she could scarcely breathe

or move

while cruel eyes

observed her –

dispassionately.

2006

A Pale Horse

("And I beheld a pale horse, and on the back of the horse a rider, and the name of the rider is Death…" *Book of Revelations*).

A dream, a vision,

a Pale Horse –

white, white against the blue black

night,

caught in a frozen moment,

timeless.

From the pale crescent

waxing Moon

purple cascades cloak

a hidden rider

whose name is known

to all.

In a world carpeted with the

vitality of nascent green

stands this beautiful beast,

this creature Creator made,

and on his back he carries

the fate of all who live

below Heaven.

2006

Lot's Wife

"Don't trouble your pretty head",

he said, "Just don't look back,

never look back,

keep your vow,

obey me now

and you'll be OK

my little wife."

She hadn't wanted to leave her home,

her friends, her busy city life.

her hopes and dreams were

swiftly turning to ashes – now

flames licked at her and

sulphur hung in the hot air.

Breathing hard, she stopped, and,

longing for one last look,

turned slightly towards

the glowering horizon.

For a fraction of a second her eyes gleamed

then became two sightless white crystals.

Inanimate, calcified, she now stands alone,

a crumbling pillar of salty longing –

fragmenting in the dry desert air.

2006

A New Witch on the Ward

They brought her in,

white-faced and stick thin,

left her sitting motionless,

staring vacantly

with those eyes that had seen

so many waking nightmares.

She was trying to stop up her ears

against the sibilant sounds,

the ceaseless whisperings that haunted

the endless day

and the fevered, restless night.

Someone said, "She looks like a witch",

another said that she herself had once

looked that way too and

that someone should fetch the poor girl some

coffee.

Then a hot sweet drink

was put into her hands,

gratefully she gulped it down and, somewhere,

a voice was heard whispering, "Thanks".

2006

From the Ruins…

In an act of destruction

they shattered the sacred spaces,

altars were torn down and

the glowing glass

with its colours of red, blue, gold

and green lay smashed all to pieces.

They left the sanctuaries to rot

so nothing might remain but rubble.

But some of the stone-carved holy faces

they left to decay there

to destroy any lingering

remnant, any trace of belief.

See though, how those crumbling statues

still bless the onlooker –

how brightly the birds fly around the

sacred images

and how flowers bloom there –

the grass is yet more intensely green

around those blessed feet.

The spiral staircase still winds

ever upward,

though, now the church itself is gone,

it merely points to the heavens.

From the ruins

the bells of Paradise still ring out

across the sleeping land.

2006

This England.

And is this still my England?

The England where as a child I roamed, picking

my way over the rubble of the bombed out

buildings, appalled by the torn houses; kitchens

and

 bathrooms laid bare - ripped asunder. I'd

shiver, thinking of the dead all blown to pieces...

And is it still the England of the 'Kiss Me Quick' hat

and the cold, salty, seaweed smelling sea; gritty

sandwiches

eaten on some sandy, windy beach?

Is this still the place where I grew up,

 my head filled with hopes, dreams in books

read by torchlight inside a chilly cave of sheets

143

on those, oh so cold, winter nights?

It wasn't altogether pretty that England,

it always seemed to rain on holidays and often

there was nothing to eat but bread and marge.

But now we must be healthier,

live sanitized ordered lives,

and even our dreams conform to some

tyranny of perfection.

<u>South Woodford.</u>

A restless night, finally

I fall asleep in the morning light

where I meet

my brother again.

We are at the bus stop at

the end of our street and I am saying

 I must go home, and

he is just as he was,

his thick rimmed glasses,

his dark, short hair brushed neat.

He bids me stay

a while and there

is a chair - one of those

folding ones from the garden where

Mum would sit on hot days sipping

a cool drink.

He sits down and I sit on his lap,

we cuddle, I drop my walking-stick.

Then he shows me a hank

of my jet-black hair that he cut off once

long ago to keep for his own.

And now, as then, my hair swings

glossy over my shoulders

as I lift my face

for him to kiss me.

And he does, he kisses passionately

so that I am uneasy in his arms

- this is, after all, my *brother*…

The bus comes, he says it will take him

all the way back to South Woodford.

I wave goodbye feeling

sad and lonely

but all too soon

I must follow him

all the way to South Woodford,

and never ever come home again.

Violation.

A quiet garden,

sunlight in stasis -

the silence is broken by

raucous laughter and

somewhere

a child screams.

The cropped green of the lawn

yawns;

a vast darkness -

Hell's mouth opens.